Lotta Bipolar Bits:
Survivors Diary Of Living Bipolar

Sylvia Meier

Limits of Liability / Disclaimer of Warranty:

The authors of this information and the accompanying materials have used their best efforts in preparing this course. The authors make no representation or warranties with respect to the accuracy, applicability, fitness, or completeness of the contents of this course. They disclaim any warranties (expressed or implied), merchantability, or fitness for any particular purpose. The authors shall in no event be held liable for any loss or other damages, including but not limited to special, incidental, consequential, or other damages.

DEDICATION

This edition of "My Bipolar World" is dedicated to all the people in this world who live with bipolar disorder. To those who love and support them. To those who take care of them. To those living with it.

It is also dedicated to my family. Whether you are my near dear live within the same 4 walls as me family, or the family I have living and supporting me from afar. Thank you.

As always it it also dedicated to my children. I know growing up with me as your mama can be tough, but I'm trying my best and I love you all with every ounce of my being.

It is also dedicated to all those I love, have lost, and everyone else in between.

And last but not least, it's dedicated to my Heather, and Lotta Bit Bear who kept me safe during my hospitalization.

CONTENTS

Introduction:

After you write so many introductions, it becomes kinda tough to find that thing you really want to say, or how you really word what you are feeling or trying to convey in your story.

As always I want people to take away from all of this a new knowledge of the illness. I want those who live with this illness to know, they are, and never will be all alone. We are all living this illness together and we always will live it together.

I want the world to know that even though I have an illness that makes it so very hard to function in the typical definition of the word, doesn't mean I gave up hope or ever will give up hope. I celebrate each and every small success and struggle to remind myself that set backs are simply set backs and not failures on my part.

In "Lotta Bipolar Bits" you'll find poems, rambles and writings that invite you inside my mind and my heart. They are in no particular order and simply further establish the "My Bipolar World" series and what it is like to live with this illness. You will also find in italics some notes made to some of the poetry.

Best of luck and much love,
Sylvia

Episode One:

Her heart crumbled as the words repeat.

She couldn't believe her ears.

Yet, she'd known it for many years.

She knew it couldn't last.

It finally came to pass.

Her heart crumbled.

Her stomach grumbled.

She cried herself to sleep.

Eternal sleep.

This one may be short and sweet, but the story behind this writing is not. It was once upon a time, my suicide note.

Sylvia Meier

Episode Two:

A false security in my voice, I didn't leave, no not by choice. You struck me and struck me hard. My emotions in it all were very scarred. You said you're sorry once again, You love me, and will love me to the very end.

I don't care.

I want away.

I live in fear of death. I don't want to die today.

You've struck me before. You'll strike me again. I'm calling it quits. This right here, right now, is the end.

No more violence. Not today.

I hate this life. I'm getting away.

You'll strike me again and apologize, but when will it end.

How many tears must I cry?

I wish I could stop the pain, yet all my energy is in vain.

I didn't have the time to pout. You may be my mother, but I want out.

You said you'd love to the end. So why did you strike me, once again.

My mother and I have a very checkered past. I've moved past the abuse and problems, but many of these poems were written in the heat of the moment, whilst things were going on.

Sylvia Meier

Episode Three:

Life is dying as we speak. Hungry mouths are crying as they'll soon grow weak.

War did this. So did greed.

So much need.

Life will die, who will then lead. Neither you nor I.

No need to cry, and I too will soon die.

Weaker, and weaker I grow.

Depression brought out a lot of pain in my writings. I had little hope for myself for the future, and even less hope for the fate of mankind.

Sylvia Meier

Episode Four:

Her eyes fluttered awake, yet her body felt as though she hadn't had a moments rest. Another sleepless night. Another night of confusion and longing.

All she wanted was to belong. Be part of something or someone. But to do that she couldn't be herself.

During the day she was one of them. She wore their clothes. She talked their talk. Laughed at their jokes. She was one of them. Or at least she pretended she was.

This is where the root of her confusion lay. In the process of belonging she had lost herself. She had lost all control of her identity. She no longer knew who she was. What she wanted to do.

Instead of the leader she had been she was now trapped in the body of one of them.

Today though, she decided would be different.

She would be herself again.

She would remove her mask of false identity and for the first time in years walk out of the door into the world as herself.

She would shrug off the ridicule. Fight back the tears. Hold her head high with confidence. Unlike them, she was going to be herself. She would be true to herself and the unique person she was born.

Sylvia Meier

Episode Five:

The crash. The soul sucking, life destroying crash. Welcome to the dark side.

I knew I had to do it but feared doing it. I was already walking such a fine line of sanity.

I know 4 days without sleep is bad. I know boundless energy without down time is bad. Yet, already I wanted it back.

Fuck, I hate the crash. It takes everything to get moving and everything to keep moving. My motivation is gone. It's shot.

I want nothing more than to lay in bed and envelop, engulf myself into the nothingness. Getting out of the apartment is hard today. So bloody hard. Why is something so seemingly simple so damn hard?

I miss my girl so much today. It's been a rough day without out her.

At the same time I don't want her to see me like this.

I don't want her to see her girl reduced to a lump laying in bed, tired, exhausted, depressed. On the verge of tears. Tears over nothing. Ugh.

It takes so much just to keep the pen writing, but I know I need to. I know I have to. Otherwise, otherwise I will simply fade into the darkness of the crash.

Sylvia Meier

Episode Six:

Midst of the night and I'm wide awake. Awake. Wide awake.

The manic roller coaster is coming. She wants my body, she wants my soul, she's already battling for my mind.

This time I fight back. I fight back hard.

I won't allow her to take control. My Miss Manic needs to find someone else to take over. Someone else's life to ruin. Someone who doesn't mind the ride, and the very inevitable crash.

I'm getting better. I know I am. I know I'm heading up there. I know the ride is taking me away. But I am slamming on the brakes.

Familiar urges are there. Familiar urges that Miss Manic is using to try and entice me into giving her back control. She can't have control. She is not allowed to have control.

This is MY life. I have taken it back. I have reclaimed it. Yes, energy is high. Yes my brain is running mad. Yes I have written and written and written over the past few weeks, but that is all the control I will let her have in my life.

Unless she agrees to play nice, which she never will, she is not allowed control. Mania is not a friend. It plays nice. It invites you into it's warm embrace, than it throws you hostage inside your body and takes you running screaming on the fastest pace ride you've ever had the displeasure of being on.

Part of me wishes to let go of control. Part of me wants to just let her take over. Part of me wants to see where she takes me. But most important, and what matters most is that my rational brain is in control.

I've already sought help to keep it under control. Something I have never done before. Never before did I have the insight to go, whoa, throw on the brakes, I'm on this ride against my will. And both feet are pounding the brakes into the ground.

I've talked to everyone who is in my inner support group. I've promised my medical team if I can no longer handle it on my own, I will give in, I will submit to the hospital. And most of all will realize it is not a failure on my part.

It's the illness. It's the very nature of the disorder. All I can hope for is moments of stability mixed into the chaos of mania and depression.

Right now stability is shot and hypo-mania is certainly settled in, and if it weren't for the insane cocktail I am putting into my body who knows how far manic I would be.

I know though, which is huge, is that I am worth it. And I can do it.

Episode Seven:

I know my illness is hard on her. She sees the ups, she sees the downs, she watches me triumph, she watches me crumble, and through it all she holds my hand and does her best to keep a smile on her face.

I know she's scared. I am too. She knows the stories of my troubled past, she knows the rather crazy things I've done, and once again I am heading manic.

The doctors are throwing a wet fire blanket on the fire this time, hoping that a hospital trip isn't in the cards. Truth be told, I am scared. It's been a year or so of stability, this off kilter crazy feeling scares the hell out of me. The doctor even suggesting the hospitalization as a means of helping horrifies me. Am I further gone than I realize.

Am I losing grip on reality.

Do I not really have things as under control as I think I do.

So the last ditch effort to keep off the hospital. A concoction of pills that makes my drawer look like a pharmacy. Multiple doses of multiple pills. They trust me enough to try and find a balance for what's going on. The hope I continue to have my wits about me, and if need be, sign into the hospital to regain full control.

The hospital is the last place I want to be. The hospital scares me. They tell me being bored and outta my mind may bring the mania into check. To me, it will simply cause me to spiral further. 4 walls to look at. Nothing to do. Nothing but time on my hands. Really?! How is that supposed to stop a mind that won't quit running. If anything at all, my mind will hasten, it will run quicker, and the thoughts will take over.

And of course I have a girlfriend and five children to think of. How the hell would they manage with me in the hospital. How in the world would my outside life continue. How in all of the powers that may be would life do what it needed to, without me there. And I know in that moment, hospitalization is simply not an option.

Zombie or not I must get this episode under control. Outta my mind or not I must regain control. Losing, giving in, or signing myself into the psych ward are simply not choices I can make.

I wish I had a magic wand that would tell the doctors exactly what it is I need to take. Something that would answer how the hell do I regain stability. How the hell do I get back to the ground. How the hell do I do this, without losing everything.

Episode Eight:

Fear. Fear is a big thing with this illness. Fear of what tomorrow will bring. Fear of when the next episode will occur, fear of the uncertainty of your stability. Fear. Fear. Fear.

At the same time you fight the fear. You cannot live a life in fear. It simply doesn't work. If you spend all that time living in fear you lose your life. You lose everything you could have or may have in your life. You lose the chance to live, the chance at happiness.

So comes acceptance. Acceptance that this is my life. This is my illness. This is my bipolar world. This is the way my life will always be. I can hope for levels of stability and be grateful and excited for when they come. I can celebrate each moment of stability as a moment of clarity, a real chance to live in my own life.

The rest of the time, stability becomes the goal. I want to be stable. I want to be able to maintain a level of success in simply living. In simply living life.

Till then I battle with it. Till then I fight with it. Till then I hope and pray that somewhere along the way, somewhere, somehow the doctors will again find the right cocktail so I can achieve stability for another year or two till the roller coaster resets itself and I am right back to this undesirable place I am right now. Till I am at this moment I am currently fighting to try and escape.

I hope one day stability is all I know. I hope one day the roller coaster becomes dismantled, falls apart and never returns to my life. As much as I love my Miss Manic, and as much as I love my Quiet Girl, I've reached a point in my life I no longer want them or need them. I've reached a place where those two girls may have been a part of my past but no longer need to have a role in my future.

Until that time though, I battle the medications, hoping the next cocktail won't make me feel like a zombie. That the next combination of medication won't make me feel more crazy than the episode that I am fighting through. That the next cocktail will be the right cocktail and the dizziness, the nausea and all those other nasty symptoms will disappear for good.

Episode Nine:

Standing alone after last night. No place for me to call home, not after that fight.

We said what we said.

What's done is now done.

Tears I did shed. It wasn't fun.

You say that you love me, and that was that.

You could not see it was too late, after the fact.

You've crushed my dreams, and my heart too.

You've torn me apart at the seams. If only you really knew.

You tell me you love me. That's just a lie.

Mother, can't you see, I'm dying inside?

As previously mentioned, my mother and I have had many as issue in my childhood.

I struggled hard to get help as a child for a disorder that was (at the current time and even presently) very unknown, and back then medicating children was rarely if ever done.

I truly felt like I was dying from the inside out and no one could help me.

Sylvia Meier

Episode Ten:

Without judgment and prejudice,

Even the ugly and rejected are beautiful.

Love the unlovable and see beauty in all. If we did this now and again, what a wonderful world this would be.

Each day when I awake I say, it's a great day to be alive. For it's a great day to be alive.

If you don't like the way things look, take a different look around.

Things could always be worse.

Just remember, it is a great day to be alive.

Approach the ugly and rejected things, people and behaviours in life without being judgmental and you will begin to see everything around you in a beautiful way. Blessed are the peacemakers.

Truth itself is an illusive thing.

You have your own and others have theirs. One does not invalidate another. Speak your truth with attentive ears. Show what you know but listen to what others truths have to tell you and teach you.

This world could be such a wonderful place. This world is such a wonderful place.

Stop and smell the roses. Help your fellow man. For no matter how hard or bad a day you're having someone out there is struggling just to live.

Sylvia Meier

Episode Eleven:

Loneliness is my middle name. Pain and sorrow my life long friends. Heartache tags along, getting lost every now and again.

Depression is my future, and false hope is my past.

How we all get along in this cold world, I'm not quite sure.

No one really pays us any notice, that's how we've gotten through this far.

Hatred enrages us and pushes us forward. Hatred for all those who hated us. Sorrow for all those who never wanted us.

I could have been something special to you but...

No one really pays us any notice.

Sometimes someone stops for awhile, to help us through. That someone consumes us.

That someone turns loneliness into companionship, pain and sorrow into love and happiness and then wonders why we hold onto them so tight. Why we don't wanna be the way we were.

Another episode written in the depths of depression. Early adolescence found my very much engulfed in the depressive side of bipolar disorder, as is shown throughout much of this book.

Sylvia Meier

Episode Twelve:

You say I'm lying.

Yet I said nothing.

You don't know my mind, so how can you say that it's a lie.

I'm dying inside.

Outside, I am alive and healthy.

So am I truly lying, or are your words.

You judge me.

You won't allow me to express myself, so what gives you the right?

You know nothing of me.

You won't, can't and don't know me.

So why do you judge me? Judge the mask you've hidden me deep behind.

Why can't I be me?!

Sylvia Meier

Episode Thirteen:

The nights are so long.

They scare me.

What if one day I wake up again to find my world has crashed down around me, or I'm the only one alive, or what if one day I simply don't wake up?

What then?

What will happen then?

Will tears be shed? Will anyone even remember my name? Or maybe I will just be another statistic.

Is that what we live for? To become a statistic for future studies by future generations that haven't even been born yet?

Or do we die so heaven and hell can exist?

What happens in the afterlife? Is there even an after life?

Maybe that's just something some cave woman said to a dying child to help ease it's pain. Maybe all of society has been raised on lies told years ago to calm a child's tears, or stop a dying mans fears.

Maybe it's all been said to end the pain. But what about the pain it'll cost when future generations find out that their whole world, their whole religion was build on old mens fables or an old ladies wise crack taken seriously.

What will happen then?

Sylvia Meier

Episode Fourteen:

Tears fall from my eyes, as words tumble from your mouth.

Was I ever really yours?

Were you ever really mine?

I question my past to no avail. You always seemed to be there.

Things are so different now.

I no longer come to you.

I only offer silent eyes instead.

No more words to say, everything's been said.

My world so empty, was it all in my head?

A world so full of love, now barely tastes of fondness.

You used to care, now I'm not so sure.

Are you even still here?

Or am I crying to memories of days gone by?

Sylvia Meier

Episode Fifteen:

Loneliness never gets easier.

I believe we just realize, we'll always be lonely.

As a child we dream up others to fight away our fears.

But then what happens in adulthood, when we no longer dream?

How does someone cope? When they're all alone in a world of six billion?

When we grow up we lose our innocence. We lose that ability to pretend. Pretend that everything's okay.

Though we often deny the fact, we all know we need friends.

As a race we need that shoulder to cry on, that someone to protect us, that somebody to tell us "Everything's gonna be okay!"

Really though, come on. How do they know?

How do they know that sorrow won't overtake us?

Or that the pain inside won't destroy us?

Or...

That we're unsure what we're even living for.

Sylvia Meier

Episode Sixteen:

I look out the window and I question my fate. Will the past repeat itself? Am I destined to repeat the problems that I have already overcome once? Or have I finally, with the help of the support and love around me beaten my illness into submission.

I hope it's the latter.

After all, almost one full year has passed. One full year where I was in control of myself, my mind, my actions, one full year where I wasn't living in fear of an illness I didn't understand, much less had accepted.

It's a change of pace for sure.

It feels like I can finally breath again.

It feels like perhaps, for the first time in my life, I can be "normal" and not normal as normal is for me, normal as normal is for those without a mental illness. Those who don't fight those demons, their past, and their illness.

Yes, I still have blips, and yes there are still times I know for sure I am not out of the woods yet, but for lack of a better word (and for using a word I hate) I think my illness is finally in remission.

I think that I can finally breath that sigh of relief and go, everything's going to be okay.

I've got this handled.

No everyday will not be perfect, and I would be crazy if I were to think such, but everyday can be alright, and there will even be days that are better than alright, and there may even be days where things won't be alright. But I will be alright with having those days.

I struggle to focus on the fact that my last major, like huge stupid crazy out of my mind episode was 4 years ago. I struggle to remind myself that all of this is a path I chose. I decided myself, not by someone else's hand to start my tomorrow over again.

I was the one who went to the doctor and said, things just ain't right. I showed him the bruises on my heart and soul, I told him of the things I had done, and I begged for help.

Chances are had I not done that that day in June, I wouldn't be here. I never would have made it this far. And that in itself gives me hope. I started my journey to wellness, no one forced it upon me (although sometimes I wish they had years prior.)

So here I sit today, confident that I can handle this. Confidence I've built over this past year with minimal issues with my illness, and more triumphs than setbacks.

Perhaps one day, all of these struggles will simply be a memory, a bipolar bit, left to the past.

Episode Seventeen:

Many days I feel as though the world is passing me by. That all I am to it is a spectator, watching as others live their lives and I struggle to hold onto mine.

It's not always like that though.

Sometimes it feels like my world is spinning so fast and dragging me along so quickly that I wish I could get off the merry go round and just for a moment become a spectator again.

It's very back and fourth this illness.

Ups and downs. Ups and downs. Stable here and there. Able to function now and again. Pulling magic rabbits out of my manic hat, doing unthinkable things, that once I hit the depressive rock bottom leave me wondering how the hell I was able to do all of that. Why I cannot simply do all of that, all of the time.

Life with this disorder becomes a balancing act. One that can sweep you either way in a heart beat. One that can take you from manic high, to depressive lows in a single moment.

One moment you can find yourself top of the world, smiling, happy, and high on life. The next moment the tears simply won't stop pouring from your eyes. You hope and pray they'll dry and stop the rain but they don't. That is until the next moment that mania washes you away into a tidal pool where you find it hard to keep your head above water and your mind in a proper state of mind.

Back and fourth, back and fourth. Can I please get off this ride? Mister, please, please stop this ride.

I kiss the ground of stability. It didn't come often in my younger years, if it ever came at all, and now when I am on stable ground I inhale the world around me, I am eternally grateful for it. And I pray the rug I stand upon is never pulled from beneath my feet again.

I know now though that stabilization can occur, and if nothing else, it gives me hope that maybe one day, I will get off this magical (or not so magical) ride and begin to truly enjoy life with those I love.

Conclusion:

It's hard to know when to end this story, because truly the story of my battle and fight with this illness will not end until I cease to be. And perhaps that's what it's meant to be. Perhaps until I can no longer form words, no longer think or write the story too should continue.

I know a lot of what I write and present reaches out to many. I've received reviews and emails that make the tears well up in my eyes.

In the end it is really an amazing and awe inspiring experience. As a child I wanted nothing more than to be an author. As an adult, even with an illness, a mental illness I have realized that dream. To me, and perhaps even others that speaks volumes about mental illness truly not being able to inhibit those with ambitions who want to reach for the stars, reach for their dreams. The route may be skewed, the results a little altered, and hell the path may be something totally unexpected, but you can do it. You really can

If you have a dream within you, no matter how big or small, don't let anything hold you back. Make today your new beginning and move forward from there. The past is simply that, the past. And trials and tribulations are simply stepping stones to make an even better story.

I love each and everyone of you from the very bottom of my heart.

Sylvia Meier

ABOUT THE AUTHOR

I'm not doing this about the author is traditional fashion. It's awkward and plain strange to write about myself in the third person.

My name is Sylvia.

I'll be 32 this summer.

I am the mother of 5 beautiful children.

I am the partner of the beautiful woman who has been my greatest support in my fight.

I am living bipolar. I have bipolar disorder type one. I was first diagnosed at 13 years old, and went through the typical denial and rebellion.

Fast forward 17 years and life is off-kilter, all sorts of wrong, my illness has left my life shattered, tattered and my life on a string.

Suicide attempt, stopped by myself was the best and worst moment of my life. It was the wake up call I needed, and the scare I needed. I took my illness in my hands, decided to be in control instead of my disorder being in control and here I am a year later in the best mental health of my life.

I won't lie, there are days that are tough, there are days I long to be manic again. Overall though, I am happy, I am healthy and I have more support in my life than I could ever imagine.

I am a writer by passion. This is not my first book and surely will not be my last. I am in the process of writing another one called "Woman Broken, A Child Lost" which is about my life, my struggles and everything in between. It too will hopefully be out this year, but is one of those stories that will not be released until perfection is reached as it is my story. My full story.

Till then you can always find me and support for yourself on my website which is my story and writings as well. Check it out at http://www.MyBipolarWorld.com

As of this moment you can find the other two books in this series on Amazon:

Living Bipolar: Learning To Live With Bipolar Disorder

http://www.amazon.com/Living-Bipolar-My-World-ebook/dp/B00CP58BLI

Bipolar Bits: Manic Madness To Depressive Depths

http://www.amazon.com/Bipolar-Bits-Madness-Depressive-ebook/dp/B00CW667IY

In the end, I send you all much love and hope. If you take nothing else from all of this at least know you are not alone, and if you ever need that ear, feel free to contact me at my site. I do my best to respond to everyone as time and living bipolar allows.

Love,
  Sylvia

www.ingramcontent.com/pod-product-compliance
Lightning Source LLC
Chambersburg PA
CBHW070505290526
45790CB00003B/1109

9 7 8 1 4 8 9 5 8 9 3 6 1